EXERCISES FOR

PREGNANT

WOMEN

A Guide for Every

Trimester

Catherine Kennedy

COPYRIGHT

TABLE OF

CONTENTS

INTRODUCTION

The happiness (or pure anxiety) you felt when you saw those two blue or pink lines appear is apparently something you will never forget. And now that you are childbearing, you may be wondering what needs to change and what can stay the same. The good news? Staying active tops the list of things to keep up with for the next 9 months. And whether you are looking to continue your current fitness routine or start a new one, this book got you covered. From cardio and strength training to stretching and core exercises, here is everything you need to know to stay fit during pregnancy.

Chapter One

Benefits of Exercising

While Pregnant

If You view exercise as simply a way to get into smaller pants, you may need to change your perspective (and preferences) now that you are pregnant. According to the American College of Obstetricians and Gynecologists (ACOG), exercise during pregnancy can reduce the incidence of:

- preterm birth
- cesarean birth

- excessive weight gain

- gestational diabetes

- Preeclampsia

- lower birth weight

It is also an effective way to:

- sustain physical fitness

- lessen low back pain.

- handle symptoms of anxiety and depression reduce stress

- enhance post-natal recuperation

Brooke Cates, prenatal and postnatal fitness expert and owner of Studio Bloom, says some exercises can be effected in each trimester to support the body through its physical changes while preparing for a simpler return to exercise postnatal. She stresses a shift of spotlight on core and pelvic floor awareness, which can help you build a more profound core-based connection before the actual changes begin to take place.

Chapter Two

Safety Tips For

Exercises While

Pregnant

When taking into account pregnancy exercises, Cates states that there are not many activities that should be eliminated from your current routines. "While most exercises can be sustained throughout each trimester, modifying and reducing them when mandatory can help increase energy, firmness, and physical adaptability as your body transforms," she says. Taking that into consideration, here are some general safety tips to consider when exercising during pregnancy, according to ACOG.

- Get your doctor's approval if you are starting to exercise for the first time or have any health problems that may prevent you from exercising.

- Drink plenty of water before, during and after

exercise.

- Wear supportive clothing, such as a sports bra or belly band.

- Do not get hot, especially in the first trimester.

- Avoid lying on your back for too long, particularly in the third trimester.

- Do not engage in contact sports and extreme yoga.

Chapter Three

Cardio Exercises for All Trimesters

Cardiovascular exercises such as walking, swimming, jogging and cycling are the priority in all three trimesters. Unless your doctor tells you to modify your physical activity, for low the US Department of Health and Human Services' Physical Activity Guidelines for Americans, which recommend at least 150 minutes of moderate-intensity aerobic activity per week. If you're used to doing high-intensity exercise, like running, or if your fitness level is high, ACOG says you can continue these activities during pregnancy with your doctor's approval, of course.

Chapter Four

Exercises for First Trimester

The first three months of pregnancy can be a wild ride full of emotions. From elation and pure joy to apprehension, worry and even fear as you realize that you are responsible for feeding, growing and keeping this little future human being safe and healthy. As long as you are not considered a high-risk pregnancy, you can continue with your regular exercise program during the first trimester, according to physical therapist Heather Jeffcoat, DPT. The foundation of a comprehensive prenatal fitness program should include at least 150 minutes of cardiovascular exercise per week and two to three days of strength training that targets major muscle groups. Emphasis should also be placed on specific exercises that will ease pregnancy and prepare you for labor and birth. (It may seem far away— but it will be there before you know it!) One important area, says Jeffcoat, is working on body awareness to prepare for changes in your posture. "Performing an exercise like the pelvic curl is a great way to start with spinal flexibility and strengthening the abdominal muscles, which will help your stomach grow," she says.

Pelvic Curl

- Lie on your back with your knees bent and your feet flat on the floor, approximately hip-width apart.

- To prepare, take a deep breath and then exhale as you tuck your pelvis (your "hips") in to leave an imprint of your spine on the floor.

- Maintain this contracted position as you continue to

exhale, performing the movement to lift the spine out of this imprint, one vertebra at a time.

- Stop when you reach the shoulder blades.

- At the top of the movement, inhale and then exhale as you tilt your body downward, returning one vertebra to the floor, one vertebra at a time, until you reach your starting position at the back of your pelvis (your " hips").

- Do 12 to 15 repetitions. For an added challenge, bring your legs all the way together.

Pelvic Brace

Do this throughout your pregnancy as long as you do not have any pelvic floor problems, such as pain during intercourse or urinary urgency.

- Lie on your back with your knees bent and your feet flat on the floor, about hip-width apart. - Bring your pelvis and lower back into a "neutral" position. To find this, make sure you rest on the back of your pelvis, creating a small space in your lower back (your back shouldn't be pressed into the floor).

- Inhale to prepare, then exhale to execute a Kegel contraction by softly closing the openings (urethra, vagina and anus). As you execute this contraction, notice how your lower abdominal muscles want to work with it.

- Slightly pull in the lower abdominal muscles with the Kegel. Inhale, relax your abdominal muscles and pelvic floor, exhale and repeat the contraction.

- Perform two sets of 8 to 15 repetitions of 3 to 5 second holds once or twice daily.

Kneeling Push Ups

This move aims to strengthen the core

and upper body together.

- Lie face down and then get on your hands and knees, keeping your knees behind your hips.

- Contract your abdominal muscles (the pelvic support) and then slowly lower your chest toward the floor as you inhale.

- Exhale as you push yourself up.

- Start with 6 to 10 and gradually increase up to 20

to 24 repetitions.

Squats

The first trimester is also a great time to start squat training! If you have access to the gym, you can also use the leg press machine. Squats, especially bodyweight squats, can be performed throughout your pregnancy. Plus, because squats strengthen all the muscles in your lower body, including your quads, glutes, and hamstrings, Jeffcoat says strengthening these muscles is a great way to protect your back so you use your legs instead. the back when lifting objects.

- Stand in front of a sofa with your back to the sofa. Start with your feet slightly wider than hip width apart. Use the sofa as a guide to ensure proper shape.

- Crouch down as if you were about to sit on the couch, but come back up as soon as your thighs start to touch it.

- Make sure you give yourself 5 seconds to go down and 3

seconds to go back up.

- Exhale while squatting; Inhale while standing.

- Perform 2 sets of 15 to 20 repetitions.

Bicep Curls

This simple but effective step is another of the best options during pregnancy. According to Jeffcoat, bicep curls are an important exercise to add to your workout because they require you to prepare your arms to repeatedly lift and hold your baby.

- Take dumbbells that weigh between 5 and 10 pounds

and stand with your feet slightly wider than your hips and your knees slightly bent.

- Exhale as you slowly bend your elbows and bring the dumbbells toward your shoulders.

- Inhale and slowly lower the weights.

- Take 3 seconds to raise the dumbbells and 5 seconds to lower them.

- Do 2 sets of 10 to 15 repetitions.

Some additional strength training variations and moves to include in the first trimester, according to Brittany Robles, MD, CPT, include:

- Weighted lunges

- Glute bridge (if you have pelvic pain or have had pelvic pain during pregnancy in the past, you can also do ba 1 presses during glute bridges (add between the thighs)

- standard push-ups When it comes to what to avoid during the first trimester, Robles recommends putting your high-intensity interval training (HIIT) on hold, since that is an easy way to exercise early in pregnancy. Robles also recommends avoiding any exercise that could cause trauma, such as contact sports.

Chapter Five

Exercises for Second Trimester

Once it becomes clear that you will be in this situation for a long time, you may notice a sense of calm and even an increase in energy over the next few weeks. Many women say this is the trimester they feel their best, so it is a great time to focus on your exercise routine. However, Robles points out that you have to be a little more careful with physical activity because the uterus gets bigger.

According to Robles, activities to avoid in the second trimester include any high- impact exercise that involves jumping, running, balance, or fatigue. Also, avoid any exercise that requires lying on your back for long periods of time.

In addition to the first trimester exercises, she considered adding some variations to her squats, such as narrow squats, single leg squats, and wide-stance squats. Incline push-ups, which target her chest, triceps and shoulders, are another exercise she can do. You should try adding this quarter.

Now that the core is in place, Cates says it is much easier to train the core while the abdomen expands. And since things are changing and growing even more right now, she often recommends expectant mothers continue to work on stability and strength, especially focusing on the inner thighs and glutes.

Incline Pushups

Stand in front of a ledge or railing and place your hands on the surface, shoulder -width apart.

- Return your body to a standing plank position with your back straight.

- Bend your arms and slowly lower your chest towards the railing or ledge.

- Straight out your arms to return to the starting position.

- Do 2 sets of 10 to 12 reps.

Hip Flexor and Quadriceps Stretch

Because of postural changes, Jeffcoat says the second trimester is the ideal time to develop a stretching routine that focuses on the hip flexors, quadriceps, lower back, glutes, and calves. Due to the changed center of gravity, the stomach tends to fall forward, which leads to a shortening of the hip flexor muscles. This exercise is a safe way to stretch during pregnancy.

- Get into a half-kneeling

position on the floor. Place your right knee on the floor and your left foot in front of you, left foot flat on the floor.

- Keeping your posture nice and upright, lunge toward your left foot until you feel a stretch in the front of your right hip and thigh.

- Hold for 30 seconds, release and then repeat 2 more times.

- Switch sides and repeat.

Side-lying Leg Lifts

To prepare for the change in center of
gravity, it is important to strengthen
the muscles that support balance and
pelvic stabilization.

- Lie on your right side with
  both knees bent and stacked
  on top of each other.

- Lift your right side slightly
  off the floor to create a
  small space between your
  waist and the floor. This

will also level your pool.

- Straighten your left leg and tilt it slightly forward. Rotate your hips so your toes point toward the floor.

- Exhale while raising your leg for about 3 seconds. Inhale again for 3 seconds. When lifting your leg, be careful not to lose the small space created between your waist and the floor.

- On each side, do 2 sets of 8

to 15 repetitions.

Mermaid Stretch

As your baby grows, it can put pressure on the diaphragm and ribs, which can be painful.

- Sit on the floor with both knees bent (or flexed) and feet facing to the right.

- As you inhale, raise your left arm toward the ceiling, then exhale and tilt your torso to the right. In this example, the stretch should be felt on the left side. Hold the position for 4 slow, deep breaths. This would be the direction of the stretch if you are experiencing discomfort on the left side.

- If there is discomfort on the right side, reverse direction. To reduce the risk of this happening, start stretching in both directions in the second trimester.

Chapter Six

Exercises for Third Trimester

During the third trimester, you will definitely notice a slowdown - if not a sudden stop - as your body begins to prepare for labor and birth. This is a great time to focus on cardiovascular activities and maintaining your flexibility and abdominal strength with:

- Walking

- Swimming

- Pregnancy yoga

- Pilates

- Pelvic floor exercises

- Bodyweight exercises

These help keep your upper and lower body muscles strong. For safety reasons, Jeffcoat recommends avoiding any exercise that poses a risk of falling. "Because your center of gravity changes daily, it is advisable to avoid exercises that would cause loss of balance, resulting in a fall and possibly an impact on the stomach, which could harm your baby," she says. It is also not uncommon to feel pain in the pubic symphysis, that is, pain in the anterior pubic bone. For this reason, Jeffcoat recommends avoiding exercises that place your legs too far apart, as this will make the pain worse.

Diastasis Recti Correction

Jeffcoat notes that, "diastasis recti (separation of the rectus abdominis muscles) is a problem for women during this time and presents as a lump running down the midline of the abdomen." To counteract this, she recommends an exercise to correct diastasis recti.

- Lie on your back and place a pillow under your head and

shoulders. The knees are bent and the feet are flat on the floor.

- Use a crib or double sheet, roll it up until it is 3 to 4 inches wide, and place it on your lower back (over your pelvis and under your ribs).

- Take the sheet and place it once on your stomach. Then grab the sides and the blade should form an X on each side as you pull.

- To prepare, take a deep

breath and then press your back into the floor while lifting your head and shoulders off the pillow. During this movement, gently " hug" the sheet around your stomach to support your abdominal muscles.

- Breathe more deeply and repeat the process 10 to 20 times. If your neck or shoulders hurt, start at 10 and work your way up.

- Do this 2 times a day.

Other low-weight exercises to aim for in the third trimester include:

- Bodyweight squats or sumo squats with a wider stance for a larger base of support (if you're pain-free pelvic)

- Standing shoulder press with light weights.

- Biceps curls with light weights

- Wall push-ups

- Modified planks

- Triceps kickbacks with light

weights

TAKEAWAY

Sustaining physical fitness during pregnancy is beneficial for both mother and baby. Doing some type of exercise most days of the week can help keep your core strong, your muscles in shape, and your cardiovascular system in tip-top shape. Plus, it can do wonders for your mental health.

Be sure to listen to your body and stop if you feel any discomfort or pain. And as always, talk to your doctor if

you have any questions or concerns
about how your body is responding to
an exercise program.